The Way To Win

The 3 Core Lifts

Russell Husted, MS

DEDICATION

To Sharon…

CONTENTS

An Individualized Approach to Weight Training

Introduction and Philosophy

From the student athlete, to the mature adult, to the senior citizen, weight training is an invaluable tool. It provides a means of achieving improved strength, flexibility and athleticism at one end of the spectrum, to the acquisition of the "fountain of youth" and over-all improved quality of life at the other.

What follows is a progressive program aimed at individuals of varying skill and strength levels. It provides workout routines built around the 3 "core lifts" and recommended supplemental exercises to accompany and compliment the same for the development of maximum size and strength.

Please Note: For optimum results, strict adherence to the program is necessary. Unlike with other sports where extra repetition of performance results in improvement (example: in basketball the more baskets you shoot, the better you get), the exact opposite is true with strength training, MORE IS NOT BETTER!! Through years of trial and error, the formula of 4 sets of 6 and 4 sets of 3 with 25-35 pounds between lowers and uppers has been found to guarantee the best results.

Central to TWTW Program are the 3 core lifts - the squat, the bench press, and the deadlift. The following describes how to execute each with pertinent information regarding necessary equipment to be used, proper positioning of the body, and correct techniques to complete each lift successfully.

I. Squat

Equipment: Weightlifting belt (mandatory step-down squat rack with adjustable safety bars, 45 pound Olympic bar, weight plates of various amount (2 ½ pounds - 100 pounds), secure collars, chalk (optional).

Position: Stand with feet shoulder-width apart, toes pointed slightly outward. Keep back straight, chin up, eyes looking up and focused on a point on the ceiling (this helps maintain balance). The bar is pulled forward and centered in the rack. The body must be centered under the bar when exercising the lift.

Technique: Grip equidistantly out from the center of the bar. Go under the bar and place the same on the back of the shoulders normally, 2 to 4 inches below the juncture of the neck and shoulders. Focus on the "ceiling point", "squat" the weight up from the rack to a standing position, and step backward two steps (to clear the rack). Squat with the weighted bar to just below parallel being sure to not extend the knees beyond the toes while keeping the feet flat on the floor. Once parallel has been "broken", return to the erect, standing position, and replace the bar in the rack with the help of the attending spotters.

II. Bench Press

Equipment: Weightlifting belt (optional) bench press bench with adjustable safety bars, 45 pound Olympic bar, wight plates of various amounts (2 ½ lbs. - 100 lbs.), secure collars, chalk for hands (recommended).

Position: Keep upper arms at a 45 degree angel to the body throughout the lift. Head, back and buttocks should remain on the bench throughout the entire lift; feet are flat on the floor (or on optional plates under foot on the floor).

Technique: With the proper hand-spacing on the bar, remove the same from the rack to a "lock-out" starting position over the chest, not the neck, lower to the bar to the chest with control while keeping the forearms perpendicular to the bar or turned slightly inward. Without bouncing the bar from the chest, press the bar upward to the "locked-out" starting position (extended arms' length above the chest); return the bar to the rack.

III. Deadlift

Equipment: Weightlifting belt (mandatory), wrestling shoes (recommended), deadlift platform (rubber mats, etc. to preserve flooring), 45 lb. Olympic bar, weight plates of various amounts (2 ½ - 100 lbs.), secure collars, chalk for hands (mandatory).

Position: Mandatory wide "Sumo" stance (promotes back stability and minimizes the possibility of injury) is used. Keep the chin up and the eyes focused on a ceiling point. Keep the back straight and place the hands shoulder-width apart on the bar and equidistant from the center located on the floor). This keeps the chest as far from the bar as possible.

Technique: Assuming this position, keep the bar in contact with the shins at all times while lifting the same from the floor. The bar remains in contact with the leg from the shin to the thigh throughout the execution of the lift. Also, toes must be turned outward (way out) to prevent the bar from touching the knee caps (which could hinder or stop the lift completely). Drive the hips forward to begin the lift, forcing the legs to do the work while taking pressure off the back. Lift the bar to an erect, standing position with shoulders back and knees "locked out". Once this has been successfully achieved, keeping eyes focused on the ceiling point (to protect the back), and, with control, return the bar to its starting position on the floor.

(See the following forms "A", "B" and "C" for recording workouts for the three core lifts, the "Squat", the "Bench Press", and the "Deadlift".

Supplemental Exercises

In addition to the 3 core exercises: the squat, the bench press and the deadlift, there is an array of supplemental exercises which isolate the development of and increase the size and/or strength of the specific muscle groups which support these core lifts. The increased size and strength achieved through these supplemental exercises also promotes the stabilization of joints which helps to inhibit injury. It must be remembered, also, that these "supplements" need to be inserted at certain points after the completion of the core exercises. This will be addressed after the following:

The following exercises MUST be done in this exact sequence.

EXERCISES FOR TRICEPS, WRISTS AND FOREARMS:
(Select 1 for these 2 exercises for supplementation).

FRENCH PRESS: The author highly recommends the FRENCH PRESS.

-Equipment: Bench press bench and bar (E-Z curl bar, 15lb. bar and/or 45lb. bar later on).

-Position: Lie on back on bench (similar to body positioning for the bench press) with body close to the front end of the bench (so bar clears the uprights while performing the exercise).

-Technique: Grip the bar at shoulders' width apart, and remove the bar from the rack (training partner may assist). Bring the bar over the chest and elbows inward so they're parallel to each other. Being in control, slowly lower the bar to the chin while raising the head no more than 2 inches to meet the bar and slowly "break the wrist" backward. Be sure the thumbs are securely wrapped around the bar. 4 sets of 10 reps is a good point at which to begin. When good form is established and confidence is achieved, add 5lbs. to 4 sets of 6 reps. Add 1 rep each workout until 10 reps are mastered; add another 5lbs., and repeat the procedure. NOTE: By breaking (curling) wrists forward and backward, wrist and forearms are strengthened. This is a time-saver so additional exercises for these body areas don't have to be included in workouts.

TRICEP PUSH-DOWNS:

-Equipment: Cable cross-over machine or lat pull down tricep machine.

-Position: Begin in standing position, feet shoulders'-width apart, hands on tricep bar 6-8" out from the center of the bar at chest level with elbows close to the sides of the body.

-Technique: Grasp the bar in the proper position with thumbs wrapped around the bar. Place the head to one side of the cable, lean forward for leverage, and execute a set of 10 reps "breaking the wrists" back at the top and forward at the bottom. In the next set, head placement is on the other side of the cable (this is for symmetrical muscular development). Repeat this process until 4 sets of 10 reps have been completed. When good form has been established and confidence is achieved, add 5lbs. to 4 sets of 6 reps. Add 1 rep each workout until 10 reps are mastered; add 5lbs., and repeat the procedure.

EXERCISES FOR PECTORAL DEVELOPMENT:
(Both of the following exercises are needed for good pectoral development).

FLAT BENCH DUMBBELL FLIES:

-Equipment: Flat bench and dumbbells.

-Position: Lie flat on the bench - feet flat on the floor, head down to start, thumbs wrapped around the dumbbells - and place the dumbbells upon the mid-pectoral area.

-Technique: Raise the dumbbells directly above the mid-pectoral area. With a slight bend in the elbows, "fly" the weight outward from the body; lower the weight until a good "stretch" is felt in the mid-pectoral region. At this point, the elbows should be at a 45 degree angle from the sides of the body. From here, employ the "shoulder drive" and straighten the arms slowly to the starting position - "squeezing the ball" between the mid-pectoral muscles; hold for 3 seconds. Trembling should occur again here as described in the following exercise - "Technique." Complete 4 sets of 10 reps. When good form is established and confidence is achieved, add 5lbs. to 4 sets of 6 reps. Add 1 rep each workout until 10 reps are mastered; add 5lbs., and repeat the procedure.

INCLINE DUMBBELL FLIES:

-Equipment: Incline bench and dumbbells.

-Position: The back of the combination flat/incline bench is positioned at a 45 degree angle; the dumbbells are placed on the upper pectoral muscles and fully extended directly upward (not too high over the deltoids, nor too low over the mid-pectoral region). This is always the starting and ending position for the exercise.

-Technique: "Flying" the weights outward from the body while keeping the dumbbells in a linear position, the elbows slightly bent at a 45 degree angle to the body, lower the arms until a good "stretch" is felt in the upper pectoral area. Lift with the shoulders and DRIVE with them, squeezing the pectorals together (imagine squeezing a ball between the upper pectoral muscles), and hold for 3 seconds at the finish position. This typically causes a slight trembling of the arms if the exercise is done properly. This trembling becomes more apparent as reps and sets increase in number. Complete 4 sets of 10 reps. When good form is established and confidence is achieved, add 5lbs. to 4 sets of 6 reps. Add 1 rep each workout until 10 reps are mastered; add 5lbs., and repeat the procedure.

EXERCISES FOR DELTOID DEVELOPMENT:
(All exercises need to be implemented and completed for good muscular development).

ANTERIOR DUMBBELL RAISES:

-Equipment: Dumbbells.

-Position: Stand erect - feet shoulder-width apart. Arms at sides with elbows slightly bent (throughout entire exercise) - place weights with dumbbell ends facing forward.

-Technique: Raise 1 arm only so that the underside of the dumbbell is 6" above the shoulder line (keep the shoulders stationary and square to the wall). Alternate arms in completing this exercise. It is important to "muscle" the weight up (not swing it) while keeping the elbows directed at the floor. Also, be careful to not "curl" the weight. Complete 4 sets of 10 reps. When good form is established and confidence is achieved, add 5lbs. to 4 sets of 6 reps. Add 1 rep each work-out until 10 reps are mastered; add 5lbs., and repeat the procedure. NOTE: Facing a mirror helps ensure proper form.

LATERAL DUMBBELL RAISES:

-Equipment: Dumbbells.

-Position: Stand slightly bent forward - feet shoulder width apart, knees slightly bent - place dumbbells at sides with their fronts facing forward while keeping wrists slightly bent inward.

-<u>Technique</u>: Elevate <u>both</u> dumbbells laterally outward from the body up to the shoulder line, being sure that the elbows are always in a position higher than the wrists. Return the dumbbells to the <u>sides</u> of the body. This is a "muscle-driven" exercise - no swinging of weights is allowed. Complete 4 sets of 10 reps. When good form is established and confidence is achieved, add 5lbs. to 4 sets of 6 reps. Add 1 rep each work-out until 10 reps are mastered; add 5lbs., and repeat the procedure.

POSTERIOR DUMBBELL RAISES:

-<u>Equipment</u>: Dumbbells, weightlifting belt.

-<u>Position:</u> Maintain a wide foot stance with knees bent and body bent forward with a flat back horizontal to the floor. Arms are positioned downward toward the floor with slightly bent elbows (throughout the entire exercise) while keeping the dumbbell ends facing forward.

-<u>Technique:</u> Raise <u>both</u> dumbbells <u>straight</u> outward to the sides - elbows are higher than the wrists but never higher than horizontal to the floor. Return to the starting position with control - and no swinging of the weights. Complete 4 sets of 10 reps. When good form is established and confidence is achieved, add 5lbs. to 4 sets of 6 reps. Add 1 rep each work-out until 10 reps are mastered; add 5lbs., and repeat the procedure. NOTE: It is important that there be <u>no</u> shoulder movement when executing this exercise.

EXERCISES FOR "LAT" DEVELOPMENT:

(These exercises are for all areas of the "lats" - upper, mid, and lower).

LAT PULL-DOWNS (for upper "lats"):

-<u>Equipment:</u> Lat pull-down machine or cable cross-over machine.

-<u>Position:</u> Sit on the bench or the floor or kneel on the floor facing the machine; establish a wide grip and keep thumbs wrapped around the pull-down bar. Keep elbows slightly bent and head tilted somewhat backward.

-<u>Technique:</u> Keeping the head tilted backward (so the bar clears the head), pull the bar down vertically to the upper chest area - the elbows are slightly bent (DO NOT CURL THE BAR). Return to the starting position (the bar is directly overhead, arms are almost fully extended above to arms' length). Complete 4 sets of 10 reps. When good form is established and confidence is achieved, add 5lbs. to 4 sets of 6 reps. Add 1 rep each work-out until 10 reps are mastered; add 5lbs., and repeat the procedure.

SEATED ROWING (for mid and lower "lats"):

- <u>Equipment:</u> Seated rowing machine (or an attachment to the cable cross-over or lat pull-down machines can be substituted).

-<u>Position:</u> In a seated position and leaning forward with arms slightly bent and elbows out from the body at a 45 degree angle, keep thumbs wrapped around the bar. (Start and finish positions).

-<u>Technique:</u> From the starting position, drive the elbows and shoulders backward while thrusting the chest outward until the body trunk is vertical; then return to the starting position. Complete 4 sets of 10 reps. When good form is established and confidence is achieved, add 5lbs. to 4 sets of 6 reps. Add 1 rep each work-out until 10 reps are mastered; add 5lbs., and repeat the procedure.

EXERCISE FOR BICEP, WRIST AND FOREARM DEVELOPMENT

2-Arm Dumbbell Curls

Equipment: Flat Bench, dumbbells

<u>Position</u>: Sit erect on the flat bench, and while keeping feet flat on the floor, grasp the dumbbells (one in each hand with thumbs wrapped around the same), and fully extend the arms toward the floor. These are the start and finish positions.

<u>Technique:</u> Slowly curl <u>both</u> dumbbells upward toward the shoulders while "breaking the wrists "forward (in control with no swinging of the weights). Reverse the process and lower the dumbbells to the starting position. Complete 4 sets of 10 reps. When good form is established and confidence is achieved, add 5 pounds to 4 sets of 6 reps. Add 1 rep each workout until 10 reps are mastered; add 5 pounds to 4 sets of 6 reps. Add 1 rep each workout until 10 reps are mastered; add 5 pounds and repeat the procedure. NOTE: By "breaking" (curling) the writs forward and backward, the wrists and forearms are strengthened. This is a "time saver" so additional exercises for these body areas don't have to be included in workouts.

EXERCISES FOR TRAPEZIUS (AND ADDITIONAL DELTOID) DEVELOPMENTS):

1. SHOULDER SHRUGS:
-<u>Equipment:</u> Dumbbells.
-<u>Position:</u> Stand upright; feet are shoulder-width apart, and arms are extended in front and downward. Grasp dumbbells keeping thumbs wrapped around them, and place them in front with ends touching. (Start and finish positions).
-<u>Technique:</u> From the starting position, "shrug" the weights upward while driving the elbows toward the ceiling (elbows are always higher than the wrists), and lift the dumbbells to just below the chin. While keeping the

elbows pointed toward the ceiling, separate the dumbbells to shoulder width; then return to the starting position while executing an arch-like movement with the arms. Complete 4 sets of 10 reps. When good form is established and confidence is achieved, add 5lbs. to 4 sets of 6 reps. Add 1 rep each work-out until 10 reps are mastered; add 5lbs., and repeat the procedure.

EXERCISE FOR THE HAMSTRING MUSCLES:

1. LEG CURLS (this exercise should be done following "squats"):
-Equipment: Leg curl/leg extension machine.
-Position: Lie on the stomach on the machine with legs extended, and the back of the ankles are positioned under the padded curling portion of the machine. (Start and finish positions).
-Technique: With control, raise the padded curling portion of the machine upward toward the buttocks, and lower back to the starting position. Complete 4 sets of 10 reps. When good form is established and confidence is achieved, add 5lbs. to 4 sets of 6 reps. Add 1 rep each work-out until 10 reps are mastered; add 5lbs., and repeat the procedure. NOTE: For complete development of the hamstring muscle, it is important to have full extension and full contraction of the muscle group when executing the exercise.

EXERCISE FOR CALF DEVELOPMENT:

The calf muscles are the strongest, yet most difficult, of the muscle groups to develop. Therefore, the strategy of reps, sets, and weights used is far different from that used in other parts of TWTW program.

-Equipment: Standing (preferably) or seated calf machine.
-Position: After padded shoulder bars have been adjusted to allow for full extension and contraction of the calf muscles, and so that the heels are not touching the floor nor the

weights touching in the stack, position the feet so that the toes are pointed outward for reps, followed by toes pointed straight for reps, and lastly, toes pointed inward for reps.

-Technique: With the proper position having been established, raise up on the ball of the feet, then lower back to the starting position with heels near, but not touching , the floor. Full extension and contraction of the calf muscles should have been achieved. Fifteen (15) reps with the toes pointed outward should be accomplished first, followed by 15 reps with the toes pointed straight, and lastly, 15 reps with the toes pointed inward.

For each position, start with 15 reps: do 3 sets of 15 reps. ADD 1 rep each workout until 25 reps have been successfully completed. Then add another plate of 20 more pounds and revert to 15 reps. Repeat the procedure.

NOTE: It is most helpful to work in groups of 3 lifters and rotate the above 3 position calf muscle exercises. This allows for the "burning" sensation to subside as well as for the recuperation of muscle groups between sets.

An Additional Note:
For complete leg development, the squat, leg curls and calf raises are the primary exercises to be implemented. "Leg extensions" have been intentionally eliminated as "squats", if done properly, accomplish the same goals. "Leg extensions" have been used only for rehabilitation purposes for knee and quadracep injury.

For recording progress for Supplemental Exercises see the following forms: Forms #6, #7-1, #7-2, 8.

SINGLING-OUT

Before actual workout sessions can be started, singling out and establishing a workout must be accomplished.

The purpose of "singling-out" is two-fold:

    1. It establishes existing strength levels entering the program.

    2. It demonstrates a level of improvement over time (usually 8 - 10 weeks).

The process of "singling-out" is as follows:
The individual selects an amount of weight he/she is confident can be successfully lifted with repetitions. During the actual procedure, however, this same amount is lifted ONLY ONCE. If the lifter has no idea how much weight he/she is capable of lifting, he/she should start out as light as possible (15 - 45 lb. bar only). If success (with relative ease) has been achieved, the lifter then adds 5 - 20 lbs of weight to the bar and repeats the basic procedure until the "failure" or "unable to lift" level has been reached. This final amount that is successfully lifted establishes the individual's beginning strength level and should then be recorded on the appropriate form for the lift performed. (See forms A, B and C; these forms are used throughout TWTW Program for recording daily workout information).

    SAFETY TIP: Spotters must be used during this procedure.

ESTABLISHING A WORKOUT

Once the "singling-out" process has been completed, the individual is ready to "establish a workout" (or re-establish one after a lay-off such as a vacation, an illness, etc.)

TWTW Program is based on the format of 4 sets of 6 reps ("lowers"), 4 sets of 3 reps ("uppers") and a "single". The "lowers" always precede the "uppers" once workouts are determined. (However, initially the "uppers" must be executed first in order to establish weight amounts to be lifted with good form.) Once this amount has been determined, subtract 30 lbs. In order to establish the weight amount for the "lowers". If this process is erroneously reversed, it's virtually impossible to take a 30 lb. increase for the "uppers". Hence, TWTW Program has been destroyed, as it is based on a 25 - 30 lb. Difference between "uppers" and "lowers". (The 30 lb. difference is used only when establishing workouts).

The individual executes the 4 sets of "uppers", then the 4 sets of "lowers", recording amounts of weight used on the appropriate form for the lift. At the completion of the workout, a single lift of an attainable amount heavier weight (but less than the "singled-out") must be accomplished with good form and then recorded.

The first after-workout single has to have been successful and, therefore, becomes the starting point for increasing after-workout singles. Following each regular workout - now the "lowers" are done first, followed by the "uppers", and if the workout seems "easy", and the form is good, a 5 lb. increase is added to the next after-workout "single". If the "single" attempt is successful, a "star" (*) is placed next to the attempted weight amount on the appropriate record-keeping form. If the attempt is failed, a "slash" (/) is written through the weight amount, and the "single" following the next workout remains the same (and continues to stay at that level until accomplished).

Once the individual's workout has been established, the next session's workout can be formulated by adding 5 lbs. to the "lowers". (Now there will be a 25 lb. difference between the "lowers" and the "uppers"). No additional poundage is to be added to the "uppers" at this time. If the individual successfully accomplishes this, the subsequent workout keeps the "lowers" at this level while adding a 5 lb. "jump" to the "uppers". (This means that now there will be a 30 lb. difference between the "uppers" and the "lowers". Note the following example which illustrates the before-mentioned 25 - 30 lb. difference between "lowers" and "uppers").

If the lifter starts missing reps, he/she needs to refer to Form #5 for clarification.

"Lowers"	Poundage Difference	"Uppers"
70 lbs.	(30)	100 lbs.
75 lbs.	(25)	100 lbs.
75 lbs.	(30)	105 lbs.
80 lbs.	(25)	105 lbs.
80 lbs.	(30)	110 lbs.

One of the major components of TWTW Program is "the one rep more" concept. See Form #5 for clarification of this major TWTW Program's philosophy.

The following is a suggested workout schedule:

Monday and Thursday: "Squat". See "core left - Squat" for "position", "equipment" and "technique" information. For supplemental exercises that follow the "Squat", see Form #6 and pertinent information for exercises listed in the section on "supplementals" and for recording the same.

Tuesday and Friday: "Bench Press", See "core lift - Bench Press" for "position", "equipment" and "technique" information. For supplemental exercises that follow the "Bench Press", see Forms 7-1, 7-2 and pertinent information for exercises listed in the section on "supplementals" and for recording the same. (Note: Due to the extensive number of supplemental exercises recommended to follow this core lift, it is difficult to complete the entire regimen. Therefore, it is permissible to do any of those unfinished exercises the next day after completion of the "deadlift" supplementals has been achieved.

Wednesday and Saturday (Saturday is optional but recommended): "Deadlift". See "core lift - Deadlift" for "position", "equipment", and "technique" information. For supplemental exercises that follow the "Deadlift", see Form #8 and pertinent information for exercises listed in the section on "supplementals" and for recording the same.

Concluding Thoughts:

After almost a half century of devising, "fine-tuning", and implementing TWTW Program, both personally and professionally, I have found nothing even remotely comparable. As a "raw", drug-free lifter, this program has helped me reach countless goals as a state, national, and world record-holder.

I thank and congratulate you for having so wisely selected TWTW Program as the vehicle to ensure your future achievements and victories.

Russ Husted

FORM B

DATE	BW	WARM UP 1	WARM UP 2	LOWERS
2/14	190	2X15(45)15 15	2X10( ).	4X6(70) 6 6
	191	2X15(45)15 15	2X10( )	4X6(75) 6 6
	192	2X15(45)15 15	2X10( ).	4X6(80) 6 6
	193	2X15(45) 15 15	2X10( )	4X6(85) 6 6
	193	2X15(45) 15 15	2X10( )	4X6(90) 6 6
	193	2X15(45) 15 15	2X10( )	4X6(95) 6 6
	194	2X15(45) 15 15	2X10( )	4X6(100) 6 6
	195	2X15(45) 15 15	2X10( )	4X6(105) 6 6
	196	2X15(45) 15 15	2X10( )	4X6(110) 6 6
	197	2X15(45) 15 15	2X10( )	4X6(115) 6 6
	198	2X15(45) 15 15	2X10( )	4X6(120) 6 6
	199	2X15(45) 15 15	2X10( )	4X6(125) 6 6
	200	2X15(45) 15 15	2X10( )	4X6(130) 6 6
	201	2X15(45) 15 15	2X10( )	4X6(135) 6 6
	200	2X15(45) 15 15	2X10( )	4X6(130) 6 6
	200	2X15(45) 15 15	2X10( )	4X6(130) 6 6

*illustrates the philosophy and practice of implementing "one rep more".

NOTE: As the weight amount becomes larger during the workout routine of 4 sets of 6 and 4 sets of 3, the amount of poundage used during warm-ups must also increase. Example:

> workout = 4 x 6 w/100 lbs.   4 x 3 w/130 lbs.
> warm-ups = 2 x 15 w/45 lbs.

> workout = 4 x 6 w/300 lbs.   4 x 3 w/330 lbs.
> warm-ups = 2 x 15 w/135 lbs.; 2 x 10 w/225 lbs.

BENCH PRESS

UPPERS							SINGLE
6	6	4X3(100)	3	3	3	3	120*
6	6	4X3(105)	3	3	3	3	130*
6	6	4X3(110)	3	3	3	3	135*
6	6	4X3(115)	3	3	3	3	145*
6	6	4X3(120)	3	3	3	3	150*
6	6	4X3(125)	3	3	3	3	~~150*~~
6	6	4X3(130)	3	3	3	3	~~150*~~
6	6	4X3(135)	3	3	3	3	160*
6	6	4X3(140)	3	3	3	3	~~160*~~
6	6	4X3(145)	3	3	3	3	165*
6	6	4X3(150)	3	3	3	3	170* 175*
6	6	4X3(160)	3	3	3	3	180* 185*
6	6	4X3(160)	3	3	3	3	190*
6	6	4X3(160)	3	3	3	3	160*
6	6	4X3(160)	3	3	3	3	190*
6	6	4X3(160)	3	3	3	3	200* 205*

NOTE: Although this chart has been set up to illustrate examples for the "bench press", the same format is used for the "squat" and the "deadlift." However, the poundage used for both of those lifts will be substantially more.

Please download at no extra charge each of these forms in PDF format from your library of purchased books from the seller of this book.

SUPPLEMENTS AFTER SQUAT

Calf Machine   Leg Curls

Date	BW	Sets	Reps	Weight		Sets	Reps	Wt	
Date	BW	Sets	Reps	Weight		Sets	Reps	Wt	
Date	BW	Sets	Reps	Weight		Sets	Reps	Wt	
Date	BW	Sets	Reps	Weight		Sets	Reps	Wt	
Date	BW	Sets	Reps	Weight		Sets	Reps	Wt	
Date	BW	Sets	Reps	Weight		Sets	Reps	Wt	
Date	BW	Sets	Reps	Weight		Sets	Reps	Wt	
Date	BW	Sets	Reps	Weight		Sets	Reps	Wt	
Date	BW	Sets	Reps	Weight		Sets	Reps	Wt	
Date	BW	Sets	Reps	Weight		Sets	Reps	Wt	
Date	BW	Sets	Reps	Weight		Sets	Reps	Wt	
Date	BW	Sets	Reps	Weight		Sets	Reps	Wt	

FORM #7-1
SUPPLEMENTS AFTER BENCH PRESS

	1-Triceps			2-Flat Bench Dumbell files			

Date	BW	Sets	Reps	WT	Sets	Reps	WT	Sets
___	___	___	x___	=[___] ___	___	___	=[___]	___ ___ ___
Date	BW	Sets	Reps	WT	Sets	Reps	WT	Sets
___	___	___	x___	=[___] ___	___	___	=[___]	___ ___ ___
Date	BW	Sets	Reps	WT	Sets	Reps	WT	Sets
___	___	___	x___	=[___] ___	___	___	=[___]	___ ___ ___
Date	BW	Sets	Reps	WT	Sets	Reps	WT	Sets
___	___	___	x___	=[___] ___	___	___	=[___]	___ ___ ___
Date	BW	Sets	Reps	WT	Sets	Reps	WT	Sets
___	___	___	x___	=[___] ___	___	___	=[___]	___ ___ ___
Date	BW	Sets	Reps	WT	Sets	Reps	WT	Sets
___	___	___	x___	=[___] ___	___	___	=[___]	___ ___ ___
Date	BW	Sets	Reps	WT	Sets	Reps	WT	Sets
___	___	___	x___	=[___] ___	___	___	=[___]	___ ___ ___
Date	BW	Sets	Reps	WT	Sets	Reps	WT	Sets
___	___	___	x___	=[___] ___	___	___	=[___]	___ ___ ___
Date	BW	Sets	Reps	WT	Sets	Reps	WT	Sets

FORM #7-1
SUPPLEMENTS AFTER BENCH PRESS

3-Incline Dumbell Files	4-Anterior Dumbell Raises

Reps Wt   Sets Reps WT

____x____=[__]____ ____ ____   ____x____=[__]____ ____ ____
          ____ ____ ____   ____ ____ ____

Reps Wt   Sets Reps WT

____x____=[__]____ ____ ____   ____x____=[__]____ ____ ____

Reps Wt   Sets Reps WT
          ____ ____ ____   ____ ____ ____
____x____=[__]____ ____ ____   ____x____=[__]____ ____ ____

Reps Wt   Sets Reps WT
          ____ ____ ____   ____ ____ ____
____x____=[__]____ ____ ____   ____x____=[__]____ ____ ____

Reps Wt   Sets Reps WT
          ____ ____ ____   ____ ____ ____
____x____=[__]____ ____ ____   ____x____=[__]____ ____ ____

Reps Wt   Sets Reps WT
          ____ ____ ____   ____ ____ ____
____x____=[__]____ ____ ____   ____x____=[__]____ ____ ____

Reps Wt   Sets Reps WT
          ____ ____ ____   ____ ____ ____
____x____=[__]____ ____ ____   ____x____=[__]____ ____ ____

Reps Wt   Sets Reps WT
          ____ ____ ____   ____ ____ ____
____x____=[__]____ ____ ____   ____x____=[__]____ ____ ____

Reps Wt   Sets Reps WT
          ____ ____ ____   ____ ____ ____

FORM #7-2
SUPPLEMENTS AFTER BENCH PRESS

	5-Lateral Dumbell Raises			6-Posterier Dumbell Flies			

Date	BW	Sets	Reps	WT	Sets	Reps	WT	Sets
—	—	— x — =[ ]			— — — — =[ ]			— — —
Date	BW	Sets	Reps	WT	Sets	Reps	WT	Sets
—	—	— x — =[ ]			— — — — =[ ]			— — —
Date	BW	Sets	Reps	WT	Sets	Reps	WT	Sets
—	—	— x — =[ ]			— — — — =[ ]			— — —
Date	BW	Sets	Reps	WT	Sets	Reps	WT	Sets
—	—	— x — =[ ]			— — — — =[ ]			— — —
Date	BW	Sets	Reps	WT	Sets	Reps	WT	Sets
—	—	— x — =[ ]			— — — — =[ ]			— — —
Date	BW	Sets	Reps	WT	Sets	Reps	WT	Sets
—	—	— x — =[ ]			— — — — =[ ]			— — —
Date	BW	Sets	Reps	WT	Sets	Reps	WT	Sets
—	—	— x — =[ ]			— — — — =[ ]			— — —
Date	BW	Sets	Reps	WT	Sets	Reps	WT	Sets
—	—	— x — =[ ]			— — — — =[ ]			— — —
Date	BW	Sets	Reps	WT	Sets	Reps	WT	Sets
—	—	— x — =[ ]			— — — — =[ ]			— — —

FORM #7-2
SUPPLEMENTS AFTER BENCH PRESS

7-Lat Pull Downs	8-Seated Rowing

Reps Wt   Sets Reps WT

_____ x _____ =[___] ___ ___ ___   _____ x _____ =[___] ___ ___ ___
                      ___ ___ ___   ___ ___ ___

Reps Wt   Sets Reps WT

_____ x _____ =[___] ___ ___ ___   _____ x _____ =[___] ___ ___ ___

Reps Wt   ___ ___ ___   Sets Reps WT   ___ ___ ___

_____ x _____ =[___] ___ ___ ___   _____ x _____ =[___] ___ ___ ___

Reps Wt   ___ ___ ___   Sets Reps WT   ___ ___ ___

_____ x _____ =[___] ___ ___ ___   _____ x _____ =[___] ___ ___ ___

Reps Wt   ___ ___ ___   Sets Reps WT   ___ ___ ___

_____ x _____ =[___] ___ ___ ___   _____ x _____ =[___] ___ ___ ___

Reps Wt   ___ ___ ___   Sets Reps WT   ___ ___ ___

_____ x _____ =[___] ___ ___ ___   _____ x _____ =[___] ___ ___ ___

Reps Wt   ___ ___ ___   Sets Reps WT   ___ ___ ___

_____ x _____ =[___] ___ ___ ___   _____ x _____ =[___] ___ ___ ___

Reps Wt   ___ ___ ___   Sets Reps WT   ___ ___ ___

_____ x _____ =[___] ___ ___ ___   _____ x _____ =[___] ___ ___ ___

Reps Wt   ___ ___ ___   Sets Reps WT   ___ ___ ___

_____ x _____ =[___] ___ ___ ___   _____ x _____ =[___] ___ ___ ___
                      ___ ___ ___   ___ ___ ___

FORM #8

SUPPLEMENTS AFTER DEAD LIFT

Shoulder Shugs _____ Arm Curls

Date	BW	Sets	Reps	Weight		Sets	Reps	Wt
____	____	____	____	____, ____ ____ ____		____	____	____,

Date	BW	Sets	Reps	Weight		Sets	Reps	Wt
____	____	____	____	____,		____	____	____,

Date	BW	Sets	Reps	Weight		Sets	Reps	Wt
____	____	____	____	____, ____ ____ ____		____	____	____,

Date	BW	Sets	Reps	Weight		Sets	Reps	Wt
____	____	____	____	____, ____ ____ ____		____	____	____,

Date	BW	Sets	Reps	Weight		Sets	Reps	Wt
____	____	____	____	____, ____ ____ ____		____	____	____,

Date	BW	Sets	Reps	Weight		Sets	Reps	Wt
____	____	____	____	____, ____ ____ ____		____	____	____,

Date	BW	Sets	Reps	Weight		Sets	Reps	Wt
____	____	____	____	____, ____ ____ ____		____	____	____,

Date	BW	Sets	Reps	Weight		Sets	Reps	Wt
____	____	____	____	____,		____	____	____,

Date	BW	Sets	Reps	Weight		Sets	Reps	Wt
____	____	____	____	____, ____ ____ ____		____	____	____,

Date	BW	Sets	Reps	Weight		Sets	Reps	Wt
____	____	____	____	____, ____ ____ ____		____	____	____,

Date	BW	Sets	Reps	Weight		Sets	Reps	Wt
____	____	____	____	____, ____ ____ ____		____	____	____,

Date	BW	Sets	Reps	Weight		Sets	Reps	Wt
____	____	____	____	____, ____ ____ ____		____	____	____,

Date	BW	Sets	Reps	Weight		Sets	Reps	Wt
____	____	____	____	____,		____	____	____,

Date	BW	Sets	Reps	Weight		Sets	Reps	Wt
____	____	____	____	____, ____ ____ ____		____	____	____,

Date	BW	Sets	Reps	Weight		Sets	Reps	Wt
____	____	____	____	____, ____ ____ ____		____	____	____,

Date	BW	Sets	Reps	Weight		Sets	Reps	Wt
____	____	____	____	____, ____ ____ ____		____	____	____,

29

Date	BW	Sets	Reps	Weight		Sets	Reps	Wt
____	____	____	____	____, ____ ____ ____		____	____	____,

Date	BW	Sets	Reps	Weight		Sets	Reps	Wt

ABOUT THE AUTHOR AND FOUNDER OF "THE WAY TO WIN" (TWTW) PROGRAM

Russell "Russ" Husted was born in Flint, Michigan. After having acquired his B.S. Degree at East Tennessee State University in Johnson City, Tennessee, he has spent his subsequent years living and training in Grand Blanc, Michigan.

Educational Background

Associate in Science Degree - Flint Community Jr. College, Flint, MI.
(Track & Field Scholarship)

Bachelor of Science Degree - East Tennessee State University, Johnson City, Tennessee.
(Track & Field Scholarship)

Masters Degree in Education - Central Michigan University, Mt. Pleasant, MI.

Additional Graduate Work: Central Michigan, Michigan State University, Azusa Pacific
 (California), Eastern Michigan University

Lifetime Athletic Achievements

High School - football, basketball, and track (State Champion). College - track and field. Powerlifting career began at age 21 and has continued into the senior years.

Personal Achievements in Powerlifting

- State (Michigan) records for the bench press in the following weight classes - 198, 220, 242, 275 and super heavy-weight
-National bench press (drug free) records in the 275 and super heavy weight classes.
-1968 - Broke the world record for the bench press in the 242 lb.

class with a "raw" lift of 530 lbs.

-Personal best bench press 555 lbs. at body weight of 265 lbs. No drugs, no shirt.

Professional Achievements

-35 years as an educator and strength trainer for high school athletics, Mt. Morris High School, Mt. Morris, MI .

-35 years as a powerlifting coach for Mt. Morris High School, Mt. Morris, MI.

-5 consecutive state (MI) powerlifting championships (years 1982 - 1986)

-1984 girls National Champions
"boys "runner-up"
Indianapolis, Indiana

-Additional 3 years powerlifting coach, Flint Powers Catholic High School, Flint, MI.